THE KIDS' GUIDE TO MOMMY'S BREAST CANCER

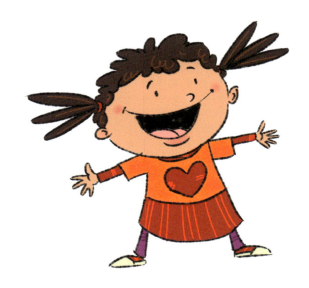

Written by **Karyn Stowe**

Illustrated and designed by **Jason Thompson**

Photographs by **Chris Gordaneer**

www.thekidsguidetocancer.com

AuthorHouse, 1663 Liberty Drive, Bloomington, IN 47403
www.authorhouse.com
Phone: 1-800-839-8640

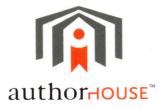

No part of this book may be reproduced, stored in a retrieval system, or transmitted by any means without the written permission of the author.

First published by AuthorHouse 09/22/2011
ISBN: 978-1-4634-4716-8 (sc)
Library of Congress Control Number: 2011913815
Printed in the United States of America

This book is printed on acid-free paper.

Because of the dynamic nature of the Internet, any web addresses or links contained in this book may have changed since publication and may no longer be vaild. The views expressed in this work are solely those of the author and do not necessarily reflect the views of the publisher, and the publisher hereby disclaims any responsibility for them.

Text copyright © 2011 by Karyn Stowe
Illustrations copyright © 2011 by Jason Thompson
Book design by Jason Thompson
Photographs copyright © 2011 by Chris Gordaneer

To Max, Annika & Charlotte, for whom this book was originally written · **KS**

To the families and kids who find themselves reading this book together · **JT**

For Betty · **CG**

HOW THIS BOOK CAME TO BE...

My personal breast cancer story is fully intertwined with Rethink Breast Cancer right from the start. In June of 2008, I went to a Rethink fundraiser with some friends, simply looking for a fun night out for a good cause. Something that was said that night resonated with me, and when I got home, I checked my breasts. There was a lump. A few weeks later, it was confirmed to be ER+ and Her2+ breast cancer.

I was 37 with absolutely no history of any cancer on either side of my family—I had always been physically active, ate well and had breastfed my children. At the time, my children were 2, 3 and 6. Being a teacher, my immediate response was to order as many books as I could find about breast cancer so I could explain what was going on in our home. While there were some books that I used, none of them truly fit what I wanted to say. So I wrote my own stories for our children: one on surgery, one on chemo, one on radiation, and one when I finished all of my treatments. I wanted to make sure that they weren't being overwhelmed with information at any given time, but had enough to feel they understood the changes that were happening in our family. I didn't know it at the time, but the beginnings of this book had been born!

Now, with the help of this book, I hope you can find an opportunity to discuss the changes happening in your family openly and honestly. Going through breast cancer treatments with young children is heartbreakingly difficult, and yet children can help us maintain a contagious zest for life that is hard to muster on your own. Kids are, of course, remarkably resilient. And so are you.

Karyn Stowe

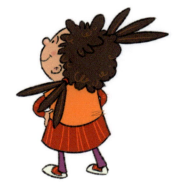

HOW THIS BOOK CAME TO BE...

I am thrilled Rethink Breast Cancer has been able to fund a passionate, talented young advocate like Karyn. It's been so exciting to see first-hand how her original idea for an innovative new resource for families has gone through various stages of development and come to fruition in the form of *The Kids' Guide to Mommy's Breast Cancer*.

I had the pleasure of first getting to know Karyn and her family through Rethink's Support Saturdays program, our weekly gathering for young families dealing with breast cancer. We know from years of running Support Saturdays that breast cancer affects the whole family. We've also observed that children are resilient and have a smoother adjustment and are less anxious when they feel included and are aware of what is happening during their mom's surgery and treatment. Cancer is not an easy subject to talk about, especially when it's your own cancer. Our hope is that *The Kids' Guide to Mommy's Breast Cancer* can spark conversations and will help kids cope with their mommy's breast cancer.

Congratulations to Karyn for her insights, hard work and determination, and her ability to gather together and lead a great team of contributors! The funds for this project were raised through Boobyball, a fabulous annual cocktail-party fundraiser for Rethink Breast Cancer. We know Boobyball supporters will be proud of helping make such an important new resource possible.

MJ DeCoteau, Founder and Executive Director, Rethink Breast Cancer

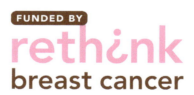

About Rethink Breast Cancer

Rethink Breast Cancer is Canada's leading breast cancer organization exclusively focused on the needs of young women. Rethink burst onto the scene in 2001 with a desire to change the face of breast cancer—to show that it is not just an older woman's disease; that young women get it too. The numbers may be small but the needs are very real. Rethink Breast Cancer's mission is to continuously pioneer cutting-edge breast cancer education, support and research that speak fearlessly to the unique needs of young women.

For more information visit **www.rethinkbreastcancer.com** or call Rethink at 1-866-RETHINK (738-4465).

Registered charity number: 892176116RR0001

TIPS FOR PARENTS

How to Use This Book

- First, read this book on your own before you begin reading it to your children. This can prepare you for any difficult sections or questions you think they might have.

- Read each chapter to your children only when you are having that particular treatment. For example, if your treatment begins with radiation, start with that chapter. Then put the book away for a few weeks until you feel your children need some information about chemo.

- You may want to explain to your children that even though these chapters are read separately, all of the treatments described in this book work together to fight Mommy's breast cancer.

- If you are uncomfortable with any words used in this book, feel free to use words that work better for you.

- At the back of the book, you'll find a Glossary with kid-friendly definitions of words related to breast cancer.

- This book is also available on-line as an App (digital book) at the Apple App Store. Remember to read only one chapter at a time on the App as well.

- This book can help parents talk to their children about breast cancer. However, you may want to explain parts of your treatment without the book once you are used to the ideas in a particular chapter.

- You and your children may experience different emotions as you read through the sections. This might be scary, and it's okay to share that you're scared too.

- Some children will want to read this book over and over again. Others will read it once and be done. Either reaction is normal and may change throughout your treatments.

- To children (and to many adults who have never had cancer), finishing treatment means you are "done" with cancer. You may find you have different feelings about this, and the last chapter looks at the changes in your home as you all try to move towards your "new normal" after breast cancer treatments.

Activity Ideas

- Each chapter includes a small project that children can do: a card, a necklace, and a calendar. Consider having paper, markers, stickers and/or inexpensive beads on hand to do these crafts with your children. They do not have to be perfect—the process itself allows children to participate in their own way.

TIPS FOR PARENTS

- Many parents find they get to understand what their children are thinking simply by playing with them. Painting, drawing, playing with puppets or dolls, scrapbooking or playing doctor are great ways for your family to connect and communicate.

- Allowing your children some time to play in their own way is also important. Follow their lead—it doesn't have to be about cancer all the time.

Tough Issues

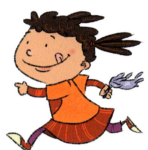

- Remind your children that you can't catch cancer from other people.

- Tell your children that nobody said anything, did anything or felt anything to cause Mommy to have cancer. They may not question this out loud, but many children think it.

- Rethink Breast Cancer maintains an up-to-date list of helpful resources relating to breast cancer and difficult issues on its website: **www.rethinkbreastcancer.com**

- If you feel you need further assistance discussing your breast cancer, seek a professional through your doctors or your local hospital.

When Children Ask "Is Mommy Going to Die?"

- Be prepared for questions around Terry Fox Day (September). You might tell your children's teachers you're undergoing cancer treatments so they can be sensitive with class discussions.

- If your children hear something they're unsure about, remind them they should talk to you. You could also tell them that "...since Terry's Marathon of Hope, the survival rates for certain types of cancer have risen from 10% to 80%."* Advancements are being made in cancer treatments every day.

    *Charlotte Ruttle, "A Letter from Charlotte." www.terryfox.org/RunA_Letter_from_Charlotte.html

- You might also check in with your children during Breast Cancer Awareness Month (October), when there are many emotionally difficult commercials and images.

- Your children may ask you tough questions about your health and mortality. These may come up immediately or several months after your diagnosis. Keep in mind that many children fear their parents dying, whether their parent is facing breast cancer or not. Children also worry more when families don't address their fears.

TIPS FOR PARENTS

- Children need to feel able to discuss death without guilt or embarrassment. They also need to understand what death is. Although it may feel uncomfortable, always use the words "die" and/or "death" when discussing mortality with your children. While it may seem gentle to describe death as a "deep sleep," it is very confusing for children and can lead to fears about sleep.

- Some helpful responses to questions about death include:

    - "Some people do die of cancer but a lot of people get better and live to be old."

    - "The doctor thinks I will be fine. Lots of people who get the kind of cancer I have live for a long time, as long as anyone else. We will tell you if anything changes."

    - "Right now, the doctors say that Mommy is doing fine, the medicine is working and is making her better. If things change, and the medicine stops working, or it looks like she might die, I will tell you."

    Joan Hamilton, *When a Parent is Sick: Helping parents explain serious illness to children* (Nova Scotia: Pottersfield Press, 2007), 31-32

- Finding natural examples of the life cycle can also be helpful. Showing a dead bug or bird is an excellent opportunity to discuss death and dying as a natural process without needing to relate it back to your illness.

- These are not easy topics for anyone to talk about. Remember, it's okay to say "This is hard for Mommy to talk about too" or "I don't know, but I'll find out for you."

- At times you might feel that your child needs more information or simply needs to spend some time with you. Trust yourself to know.

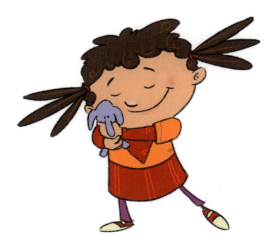

MOMMY HAS AN OPERATION

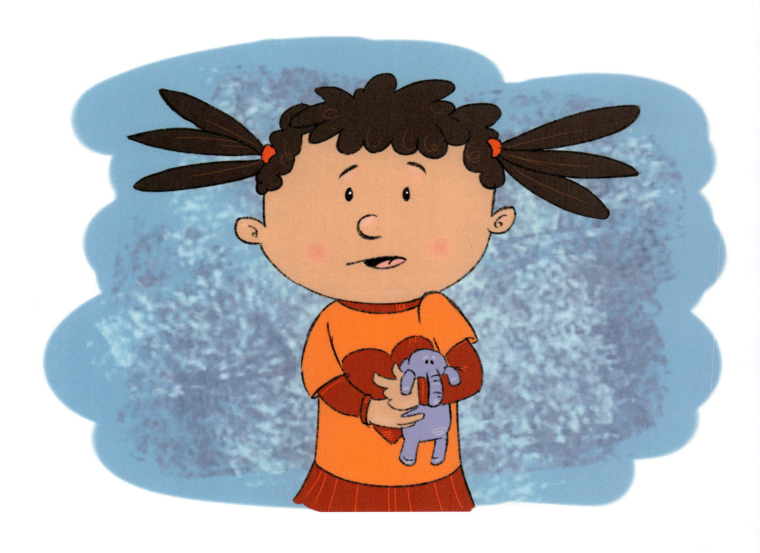

Things are changing at our house. Mommy is going to a lot of appointments and my babysitter is over all the time.

Something is going on.

Mommy tells me the doctors found a lump in her breast called **breast cancer**.

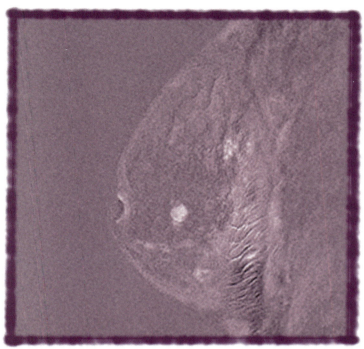

Medical image of a breast with a lump

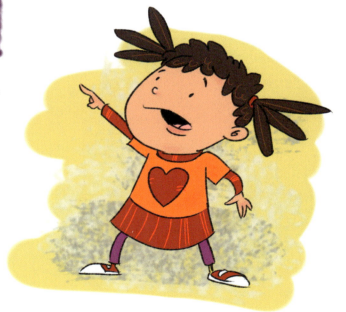

Breast cancer starts when **cells**, the tiny building blocks of our bodies, don't grow the right way and make a lump. Mommy is going to the hospital for an **operation** to take the lump out of her breast.

On the day of the operation, Mommy packs her bag and Daddy drives her to the hospital. Mommy will stay in the hospital until the doctors say she is well enough to come home. Grandma and Grandpa are staying with me while Daddy helps Mommy at the hospital.

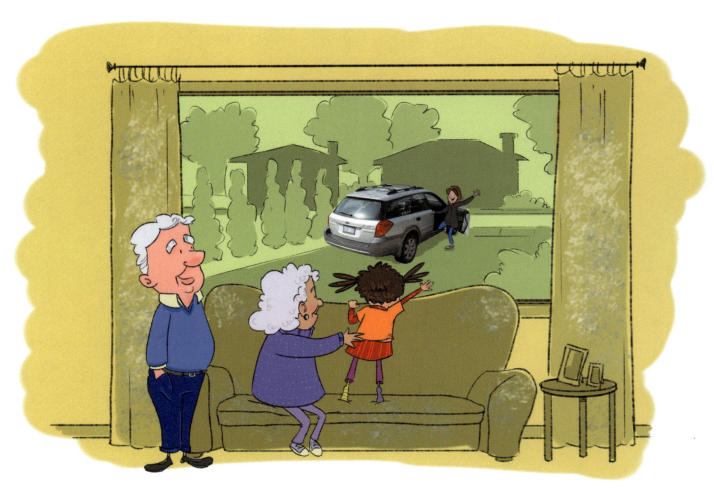

It feels different without Mommy at home, but Grandma and Grandpa let me have ice cream for dessert. Then we work together to make a beautiful card for Mommy.

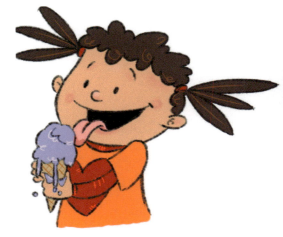

Mommy and Daddy go to meet her **surgeon**. That's a fancy name for a doctor who does operations. He says they are going to give Mommy some sleeping medicine so the operation won't hurt. Then, the surgeon will make an opening on her breast and take out the cancer.

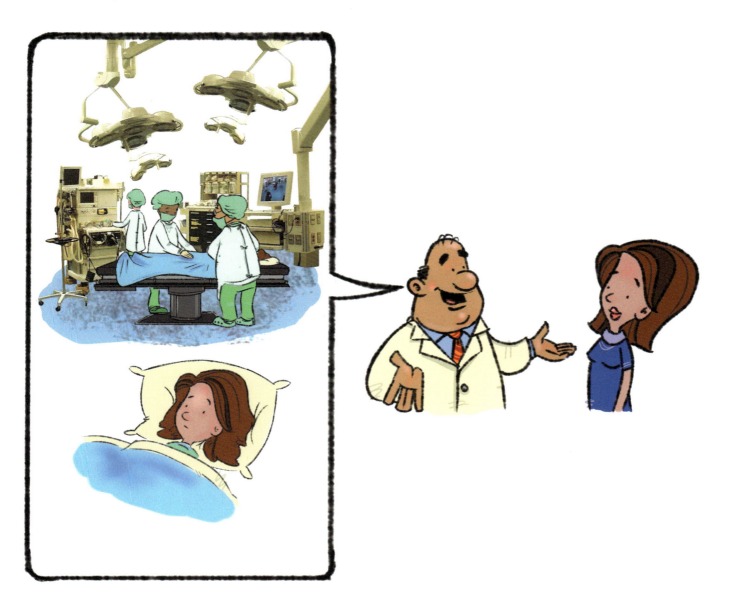

After the operation, Mommy will wake up and not remember any of it! When she comes home, she will be tired and sore. I'll need to give Mommy gentle hugs for a few weeks.

When Mommy comes home from the hospital, I run to give her the card I made.

She loves it.

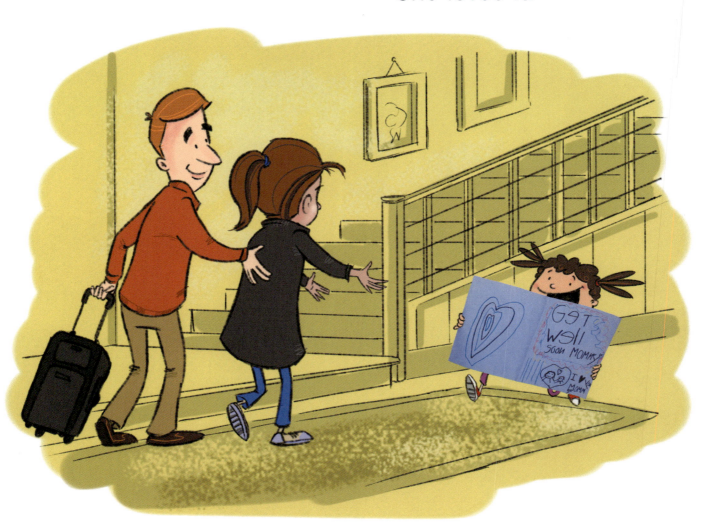

I give her a gentle hug, and then she rests in bed. I bring my stuffed animals to play quietly beside her.

Because of the operation, Mommy has a big bandage covering her chest. Under the bandage there is a mark called a **scar**. This is where the surgeon made the opening to remove the cancer. She says it's sore right now but it's going to get better every day.

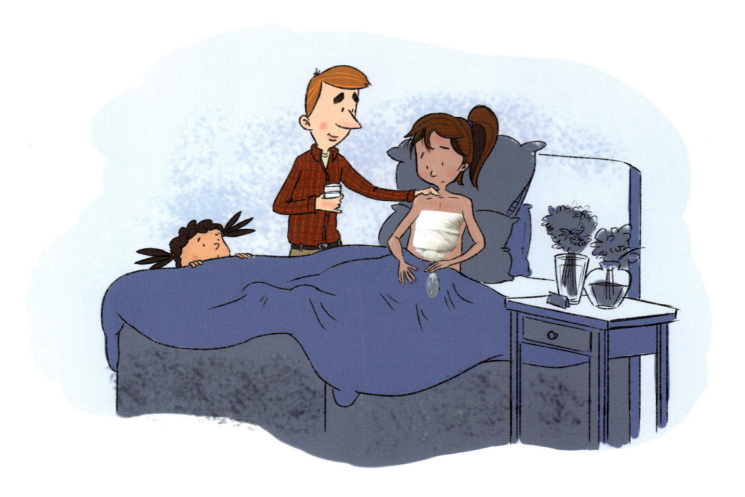

Mommy's friends bring meals so Mommy and Daddy don't have to cook. That way, Mommy can just get better and spend time with us. Mommy and Daddy say that I can always ask them any questions I have about breast cancer.

After a few days at home, Mommy is feeling better and we can sit and play together again. Finally, Mommy gets the bandages off and can wrap her arms around me for the biggest hug ever.

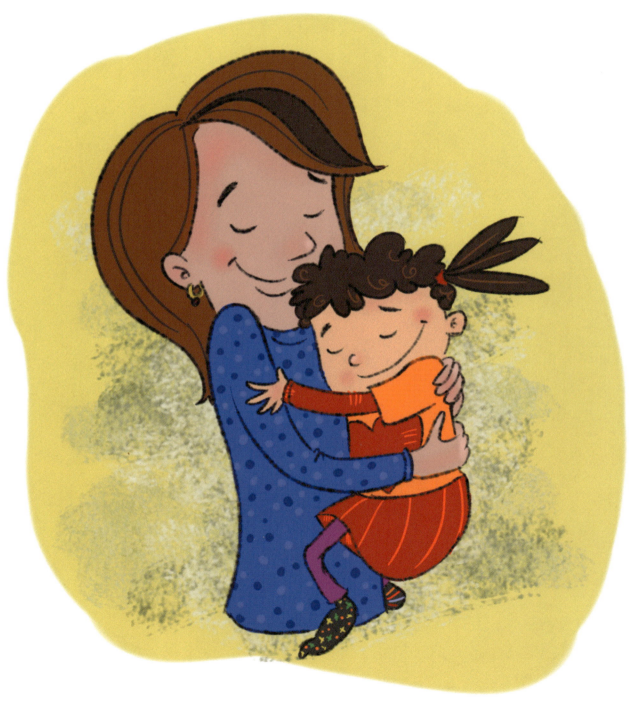

And it feels great!

MOMMY STARTS CHEMO

Things are changing at our house. Mommy is going to a lot of appointments and my babysitter is over all the time.

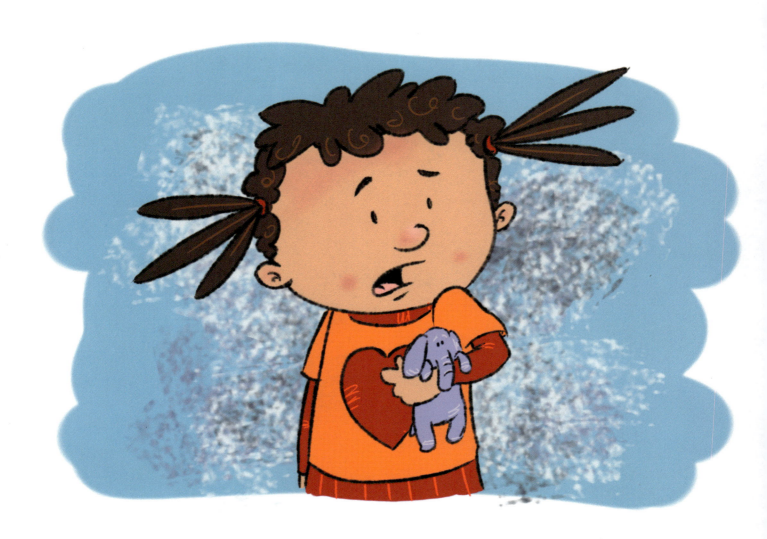

Something is going on.

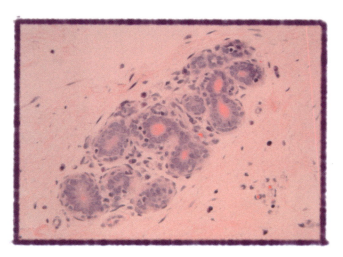
Normal breast cells

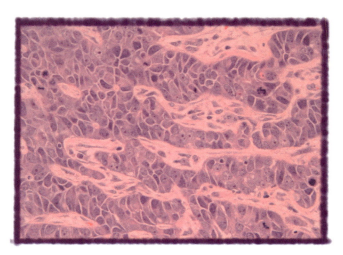
Breast cancer cells

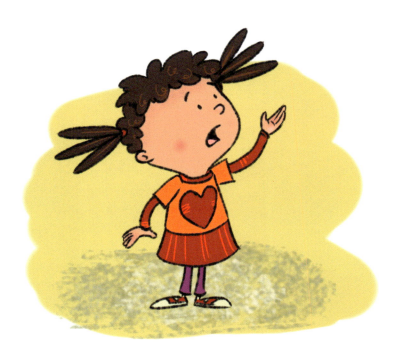

Mommy tells me the doctors found a lump in her breast called **breast cancer**. Breast cancer starts when **cells**, the tiny building blocks of our bodies, don't grow the right way and make a lump. The doctors say that Mommy is going to start taking a medicine to help fight the cancer. This medicine is called **chemotherapy**—but most people just call it **chemo**. Mommy will get chemo at the hospital.

Chemo medicine is very strong so it can destroy the unhealthy cancer cells. Chemo can also destroy healthy cells, and it might make Mommy feel sick sometimes. Mommy doesn't want to feel sick, but the doctors say that chemo can make the cancer go away. That's important.

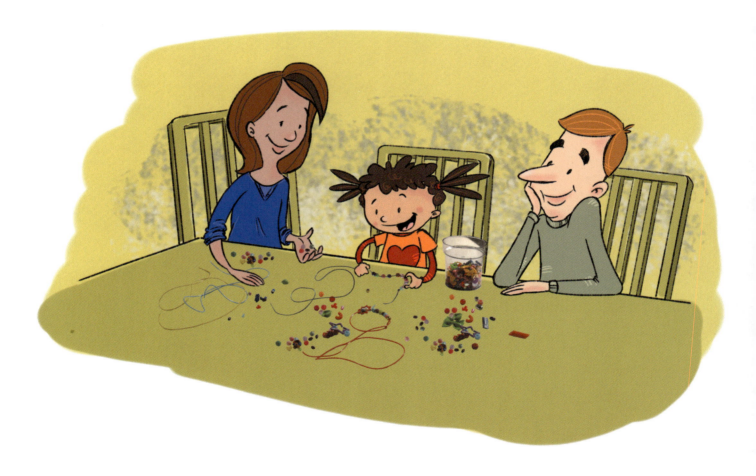

Kids can't come to chemo appointments, so we make a special necklace together. Mommy will wear it to every chemo appointment. Each time she goes, we'll add more beads.

Mommy gets her blood tested at the hospital so her **oncologist** can make sure her body is strong enough for chemo. An oncologist is a fancy name for the doctor who figures out what chemo medicine Mommy should take. She asks Mommy how she is feeling and answers all of her questions, just like Mommy and Daddy try to answer mine.

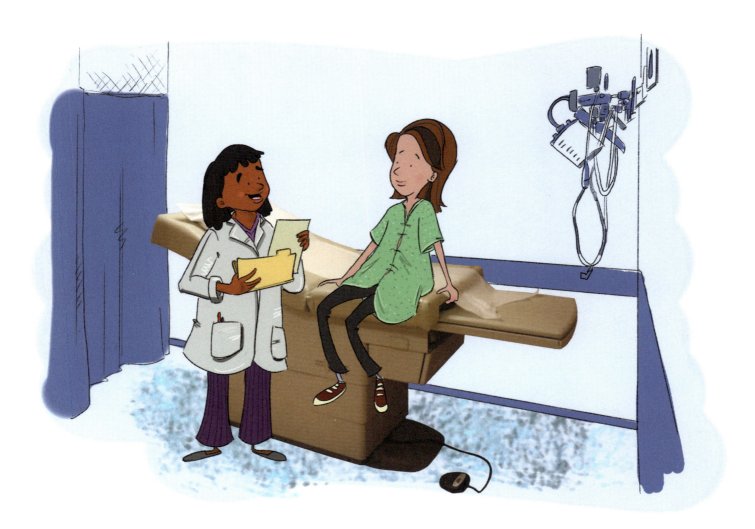

When Mommy goes for her first chemo treatment, she wears her new colourful necklace. At the hospital, she sits in a chair, and the nurses wrap her up in cozy, warm blankets. Then the nurses give Mommy the chemo medicine through **I.V. (or intravenous)** tubes.

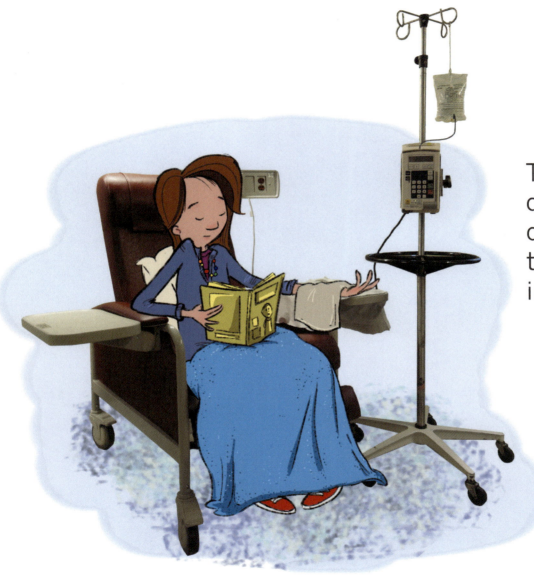

The medicine drips slowly down the I.V. tubes and into Mommy.

She says it doesn't hurt much, but it's a little boring to sit there all that time. Someone usually goes with her to keep her company. They have a snack together or Mommy has a quick nap.

After Mommy gets home from chemo, she feels a little yucky and needs to rest in bed. I go to my friend's house to play. When I get home, Mommy is still sleeping, so I work quietly on a puzzle in my room. At dinnertime, Mommy takes a long time to come to the table for dinner, and she only eats five crackers!

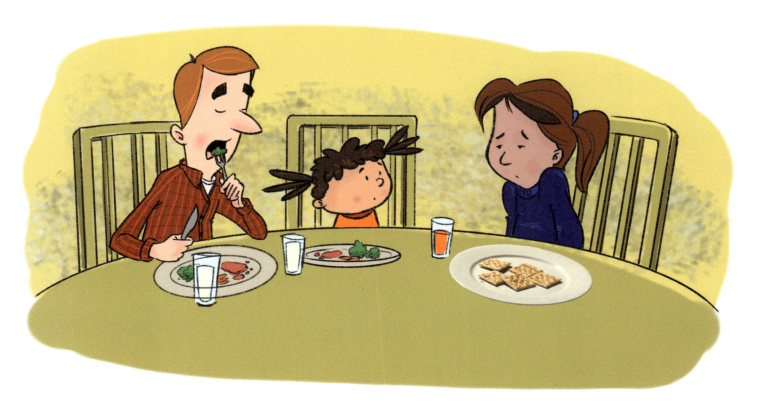

I wonder if Daddy will let her have dessert, but Mommy says she's not hungry right now.

After a few days, Mommy feels better, and I can read books on the bed beside her.

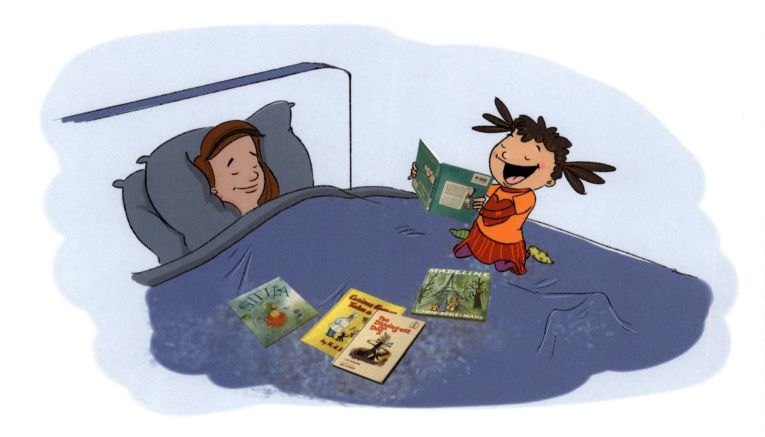

Soon Mommy feels well enough to walk me to school again. She tells me she'll have some days when she'll feel well and other days when she won't. She'll also have to go back to the hospital for more chemo in a couple of weeks.

Then Mommy says the most surprising thing.

She says that chemo makes your hair fall out!

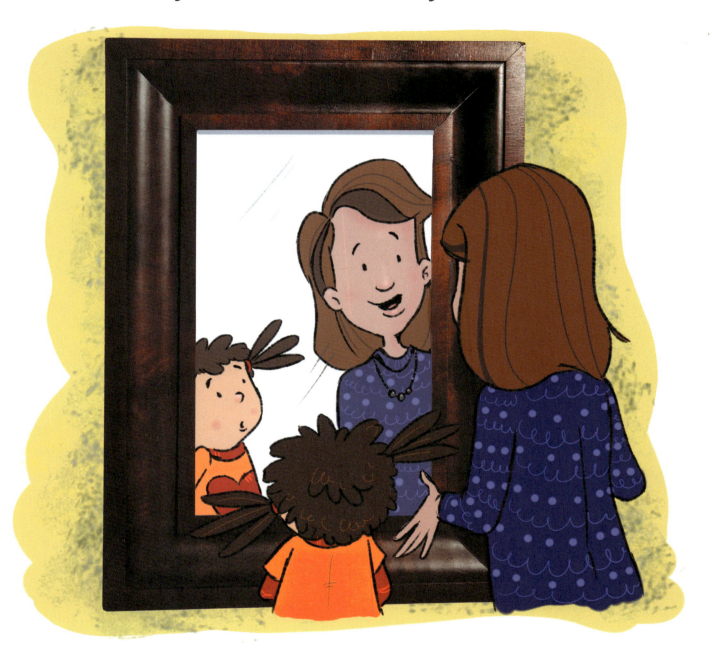

Mommy is going to be bald! I look at Mommy's hair and try to imagine her without it, but I can't.

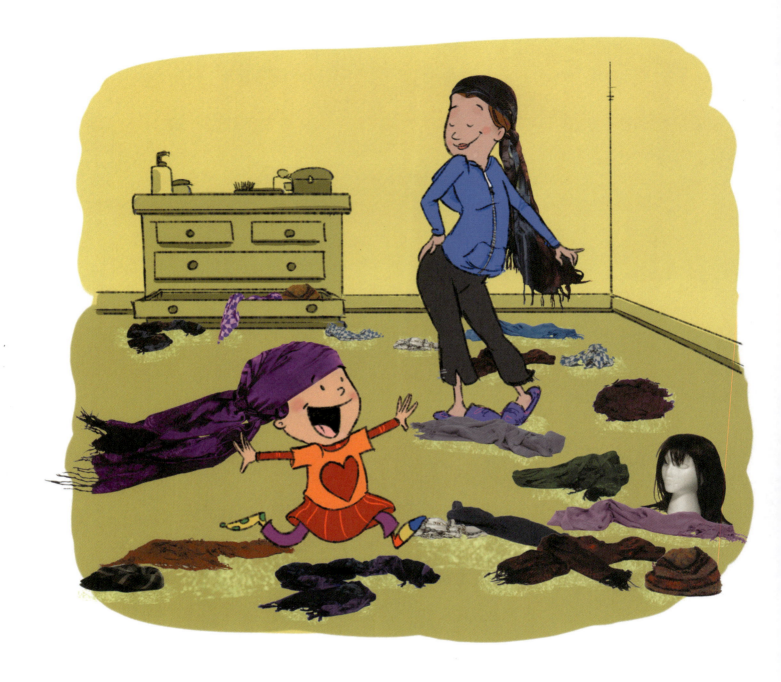

Mommy shows me all the cozy hats and colourful scarves she'll wear when her hair falls out. I try them on and play dress-up with Mommy. She even has a wig that looks just like real hair. She can wear it until her hair grows back after she's finished chemo.

Soon enough, Mommy shows me how her hair comes out when she tugs on it.

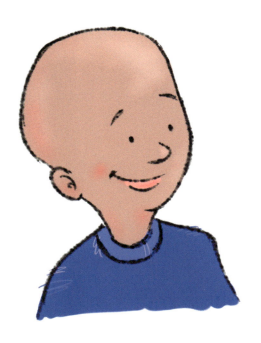

A few days later, Mommy walks into the kitchen and: Mommy is bald!

All day I stare at her.

She looks different.

But once we start laughing and playing, I get used to how Mommy looks. I realize it doesn't matter if she has hair or not.

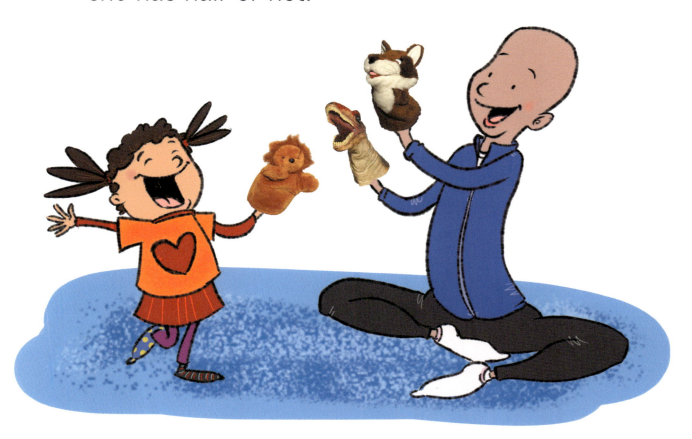

She's still my Mommy.

While Mommy is taking chemo, she feels pretty sick sometimes. Our friends and family really help out!

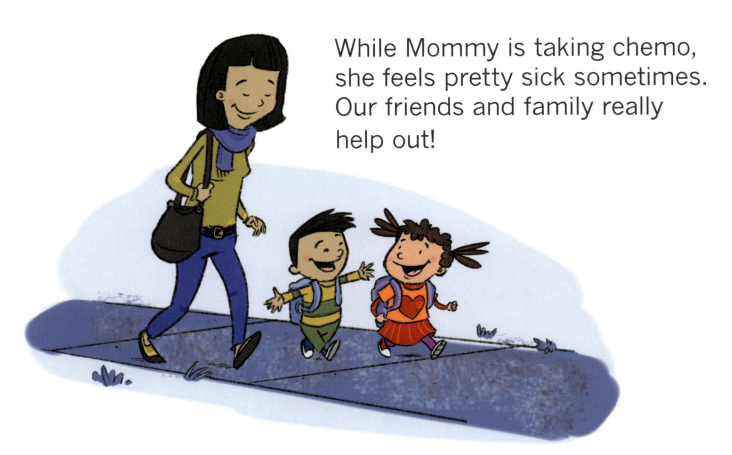

Some days, friends pick me up from school, or my babysitter comes over to play with me in the afternoon. Sometimes I go to Grandma and Grandpa's house for sleepovers.

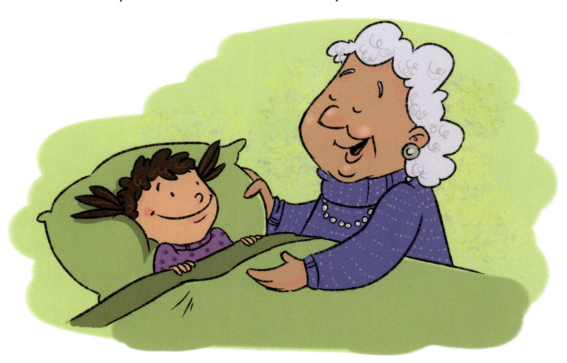

Other friends drop off meals so Mommy and Daddy don't have to cook—the smell of food cooking gives Mommy a tummy ache.

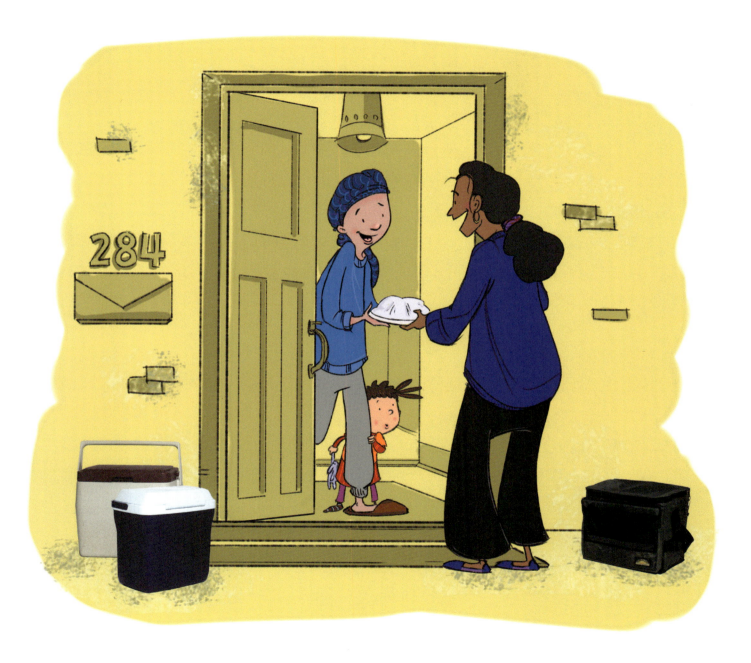

Daddy and I make a list of things I can do to help too, like clearing the dishes from the table when we're finished dinner.

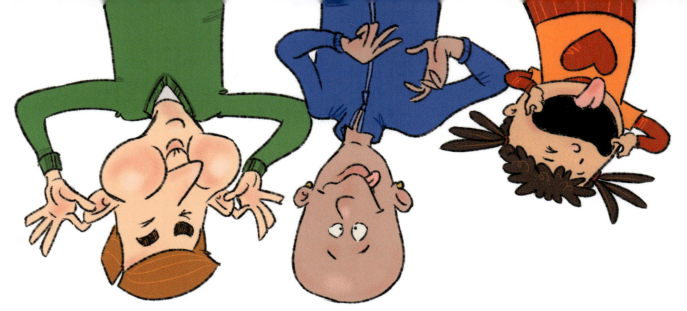

It feels like chemo takes a long time to be over. Finally, Mommy's necklace is long and beautiful, and she wears it to her last chemo appointment. Everybody cheered as Mommy left the chemo room. Even though we're excited that Mommy is finished chemo, she still feels tired. She'll feel better every day, but it will take a little while.

We decide to take some pictures of our family so we can remember what Mommy looks like with no hair. We make silly faces, mad faces and serious faces. Then we make an "I'm-so-happy-chemo-is-over" face. That's the one we put on the fridge to remember when our family got through Mommy's chemo.

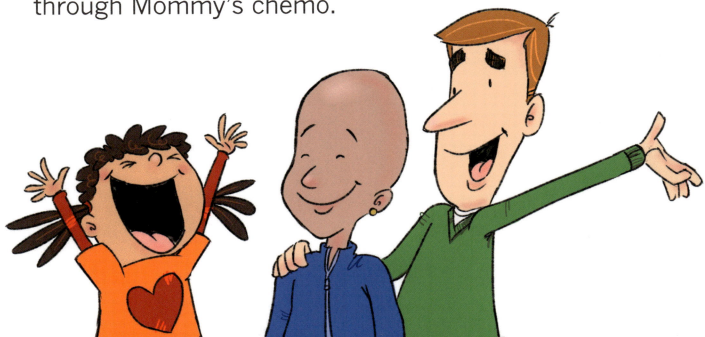

MOMMY STARTS RADIATION

Things are changing at our house. Mommy is going to a lot of appointments and my babysitter is over all the time.

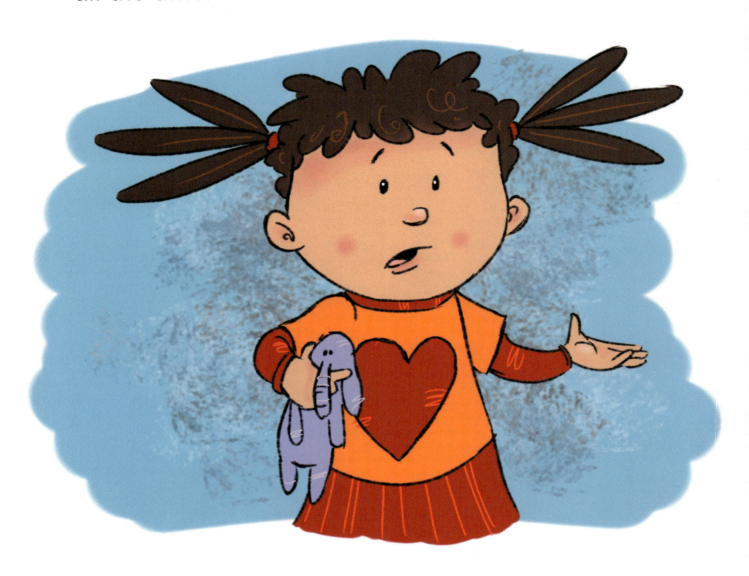

Something is going on.

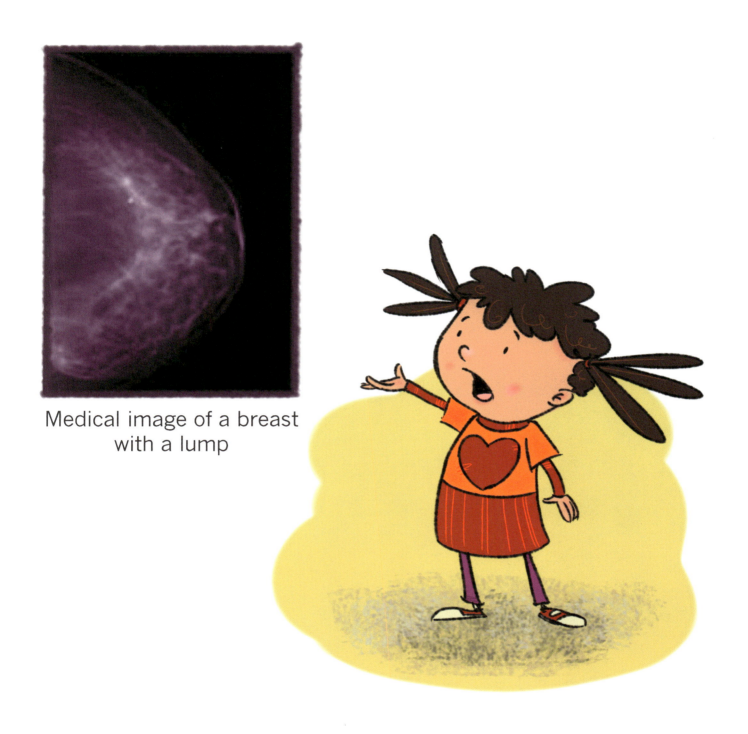

Medical image of a breast with a lump

Mommy tells me the doctors found a lump in her breast called **breast cancer**. Breast cancer starts when **cells**, the tiny building blocks of our bodies, don't grow the right way and make a lump.

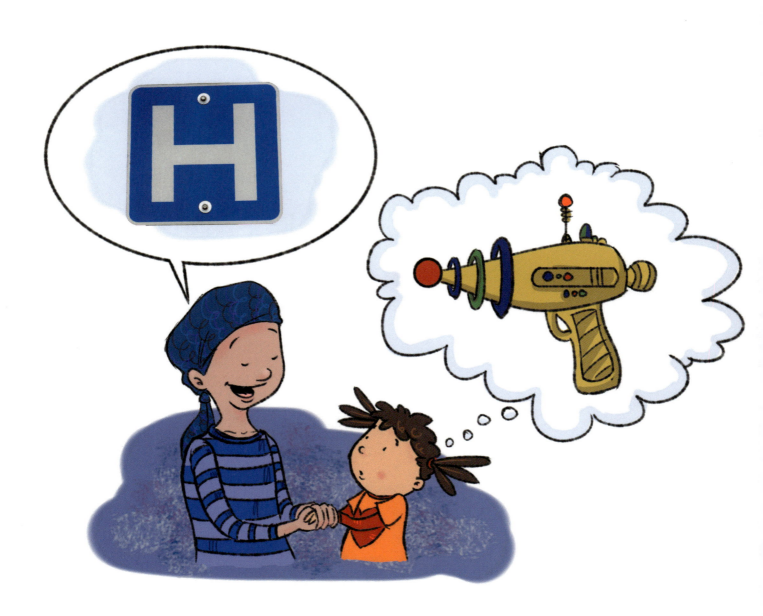

Mommy says she'll be going to the hospital for something called **radiation**. Radiation is a way to zap the cancer in her breast by using invisible energy rays. She'll have to go every day during the week but gets to take a break on weekends.

Because Mommy will have radiation for a few weeks, we make a big calendar to mark off all the radiation appointments. We'll add colourful stickers as we count down the days until it's done.

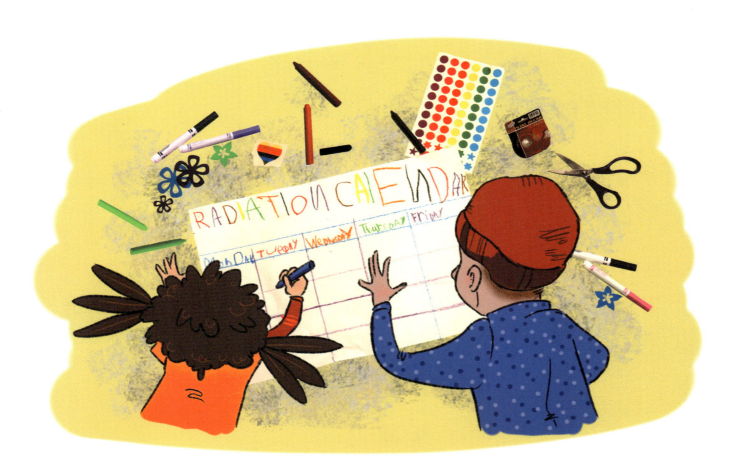

When Mommy arrives at the hospital for her radiation appointments, she changes into a gown and sits in the waiting room.

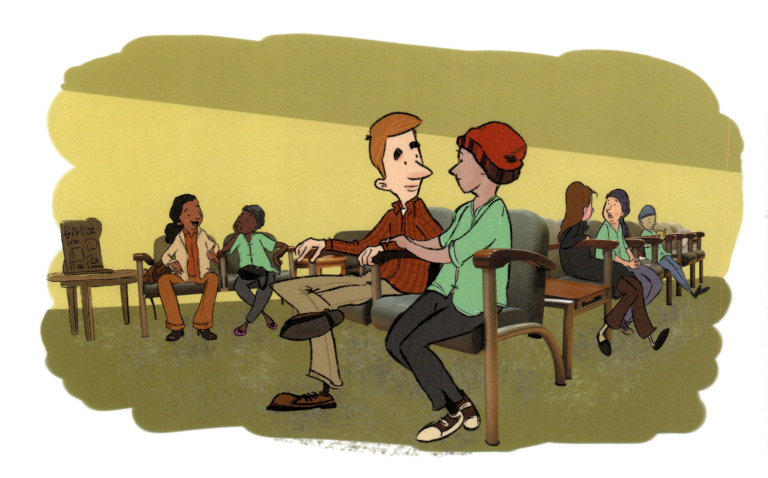

There are lots of other people waiting for their turn to have radiation too. Sometimes Daddy or one of Mommy's friends goes with her to keep her company.

When it's Mommy's turn, she goes into a room with a big machine.

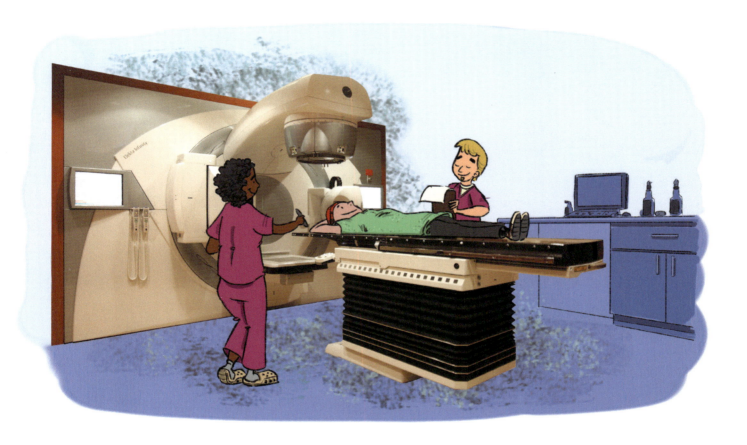

She lies down on a table with her arm over her head, and the **radiation specialists** take some measurements. They give Mommy some little, blue freckle tattoos so they can point the radiation machine to the same spot every single day.

Then, everyone leaves the room and the big machine moves around Mommy to aim the radiation at her chest.

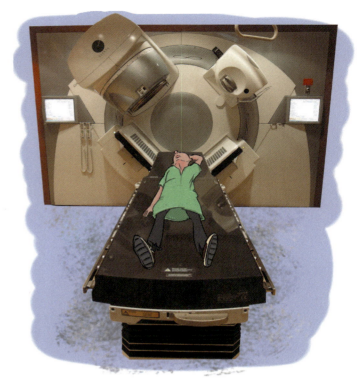

It only takes a minute or two, and she doesn't feel anything—although Mommy says her skin might get red and sore, like a sunburn, after a while.

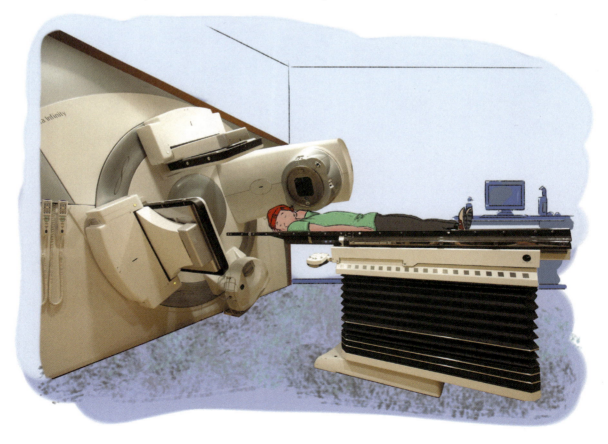

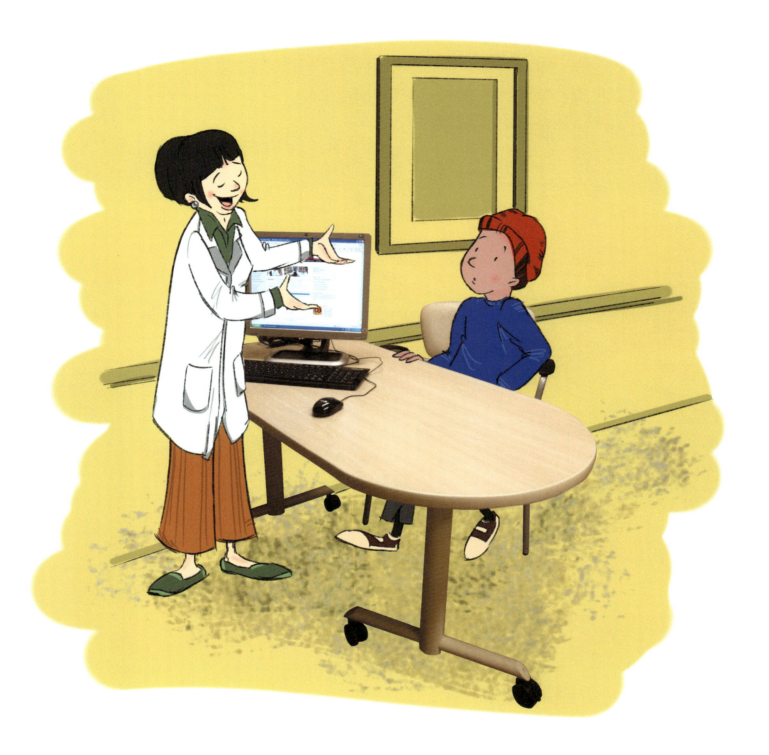

When Mommy is at the hospital, sometimes she sees her **radiation oncologist**, which is a fancy name for the doctor who makes sure the radiation treatments are designed just right for Mommy. The radiation oncologist answers all of Mommy's questions.

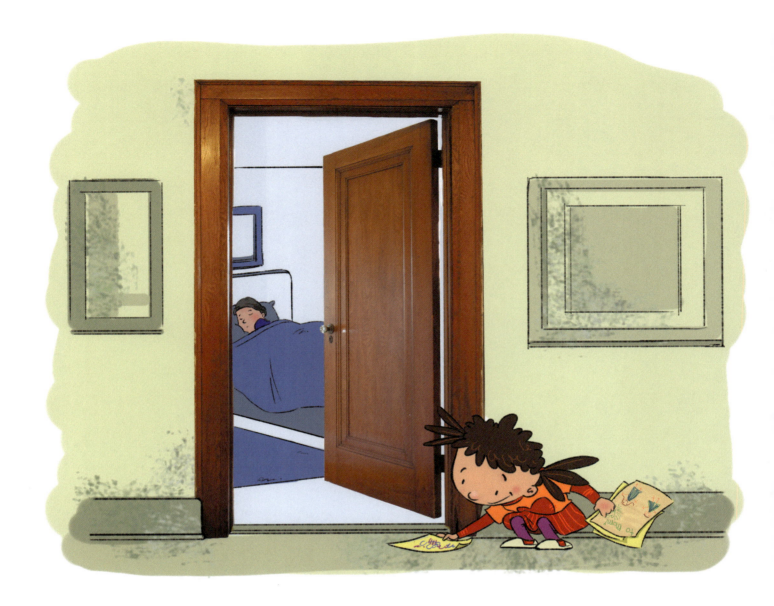

Since Mommy goes to her radiation appointments so often, she can't always pick me up from school. Some days I play at a friend's house, and other days my babysitter picks me up. Mommy also says radiation can make her feel tired. Sometimes while she naps in the afternoon, I draw her pictures and slide them under the door.

After every radiation appointment, we add a sticker to our calendar. When it's almost full, Mommy says we need to figure out a funny way to hug for a while because her chest is getting sore. We decide to rub noses instead, but we always end up giggling.

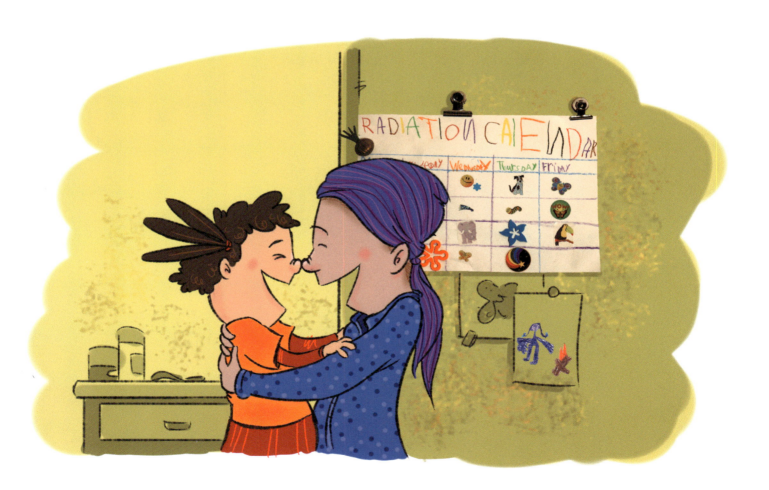

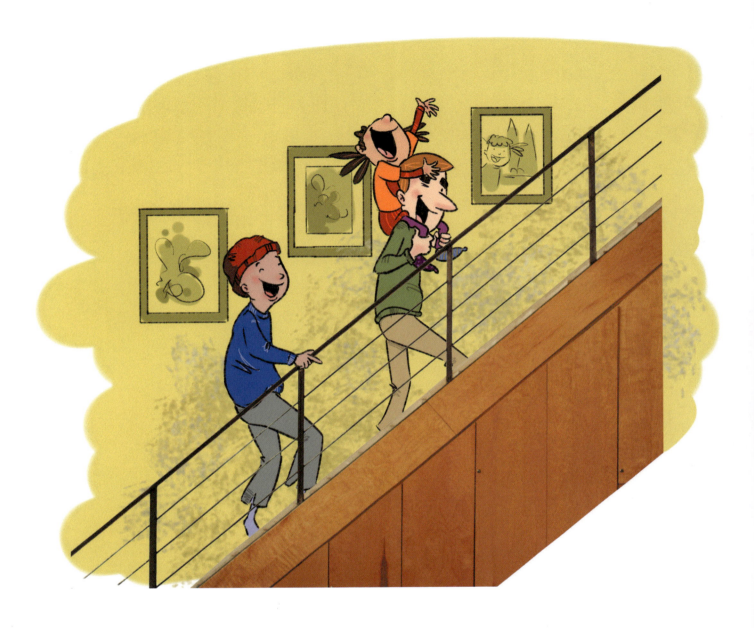

Finally, after Mommy's last radiation appointment, she says good-bye to the nurses and everyone who helped her. When Mommy gets home, we clap as we put the biggest sticker on the last day of our calendar. Mommy says she's looking forward to walking me to school again. That night, we make up lots of silly songs—I even make up a "Finished Radiation" song. We laugh as we sing "Mommy's finished radiation! Now it's time for celebration!" as we climb the stairs to bed.

MOMMY IS FINISHED BREAST CANCER TREATMENTS

A lot has changed for our family since Mommy had breast cancer. And Mommy and Daddy say there will be a few more changes, even though Mommy has finished her treatments.

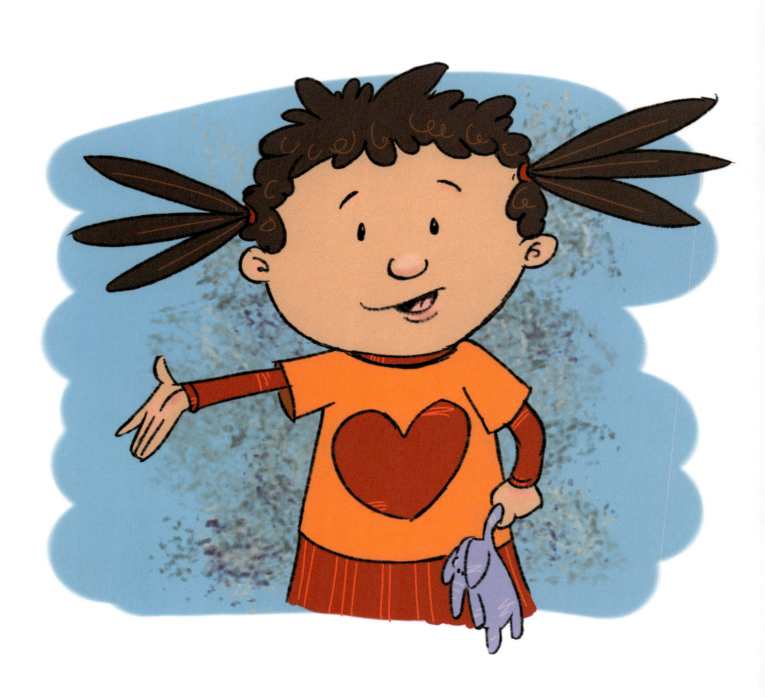

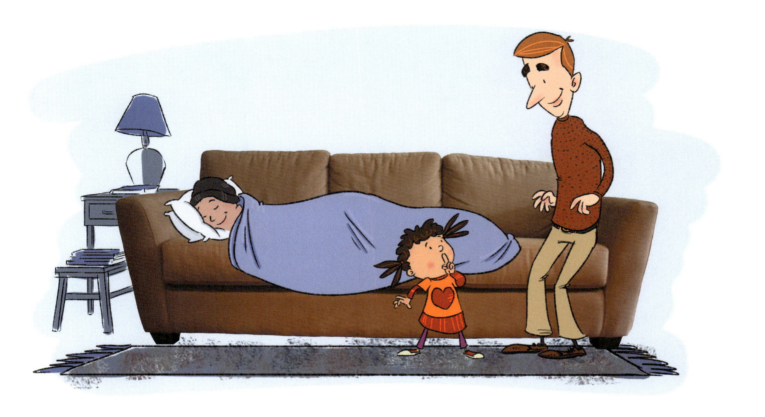

Mommy still visits the doctor, but not as often as before. She has more energy and feels better, but some days she still needs to have a nap.

Even though Mommy laughs and plays more now, sometimes she might feel sad and worried after having breast cancer—but that's normal, and every day gets better.

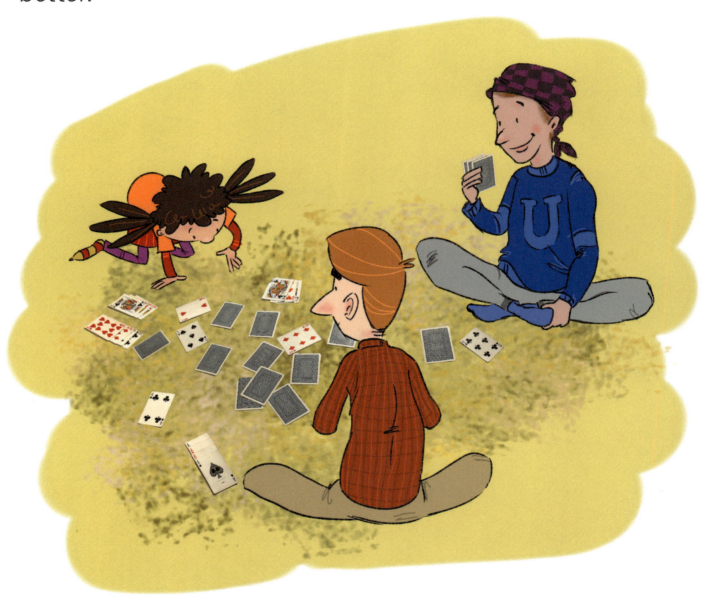

Some people call her a "Breast Cancer Survivor," but I still call her Mommy.

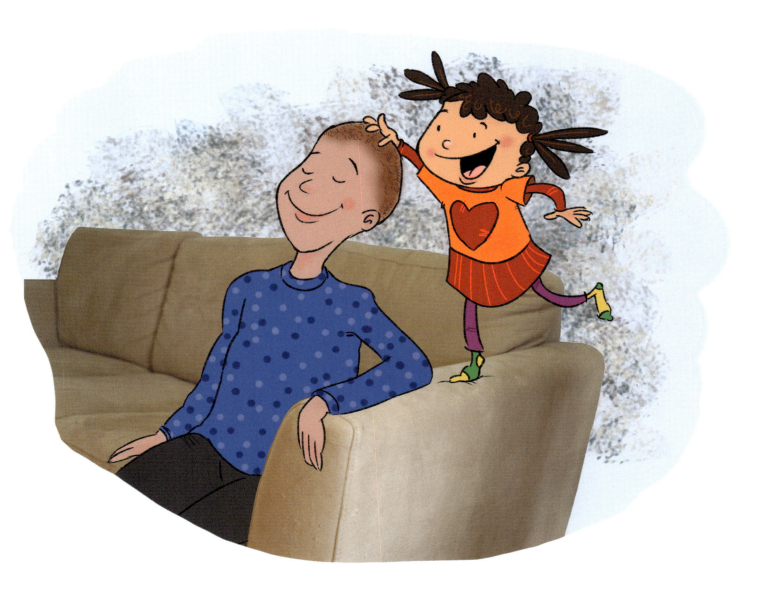

Mommy's hair is growing back too—I like to rub it because it feels a little tickly. Mommy goes out without a wig or a scarf all the time now!

Mommy and Daddy say it's important that we eat lots of healthy food—especially fruits and vegetables—to help keep our bodies strong. Carrots are my favourite vegetable, and I promised Mommy I'd even try some new ones...

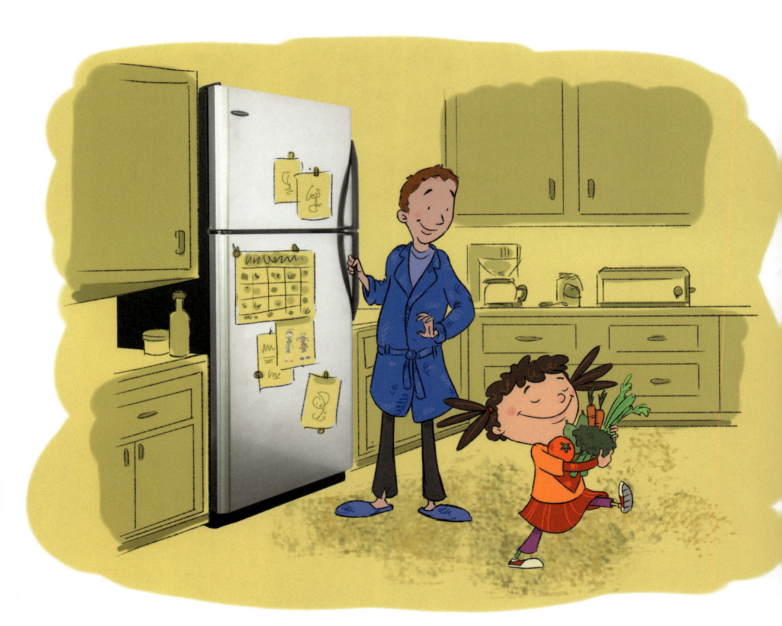

...but I'll have to work up to Brussels sprouts!

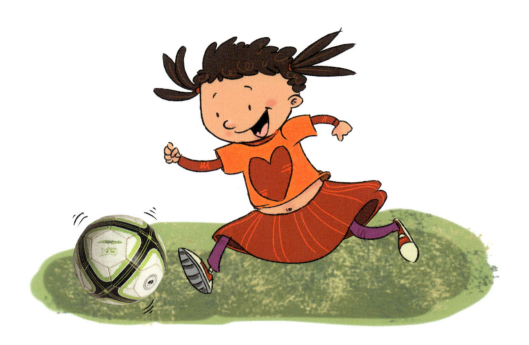

We're also exercising together to help keep our bodies fit. Mommy is starting yoga, and I'm playing soccer. On weekends, our whole family goes to the park for a bike ride.

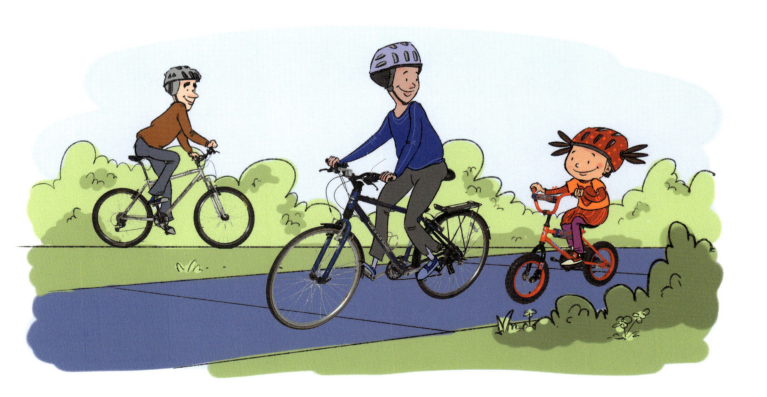

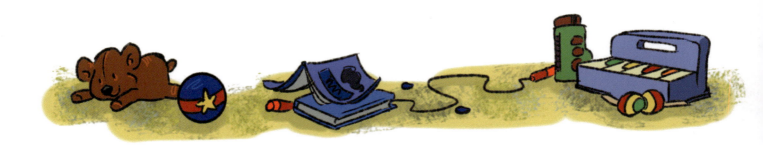

Everyone helps around the house a little bit more. I tidy up the toys and put my clothes in the laundry at the end of the day.

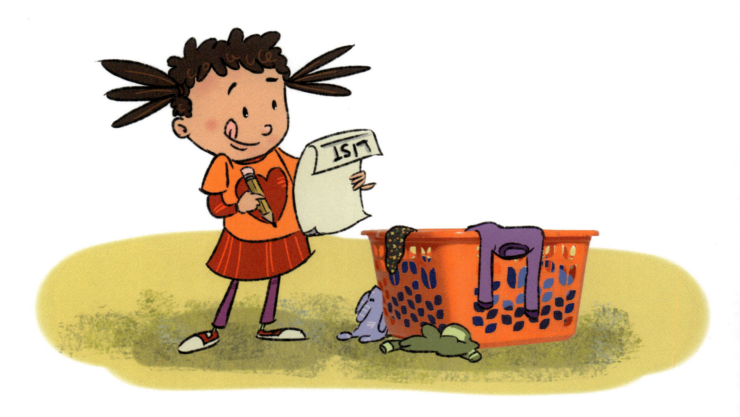

We make a list of responsibilities so everyone can do their part for our family team. I also know that if I ever have a question about breast cancer, I can always ask Mommy and Daddy.

This year, we realized how important friends and family are to help each other through tough times. Our family even decided to raise money for breast cancer charities. Mommy says the money helps scientists and doctors find new ways to help people with cancer. Hopefully they can make it easier for other families if their mommies are having breast cancer treatments too.

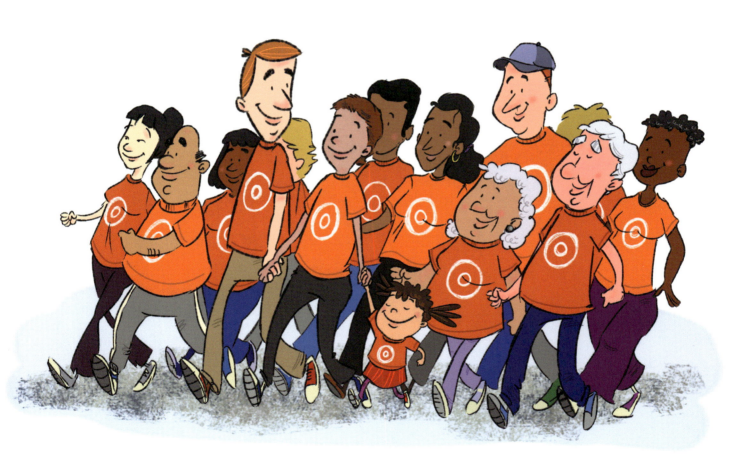

And maybe one day, they'll figure out a way to make sure that no one will ever get breast cancer again.

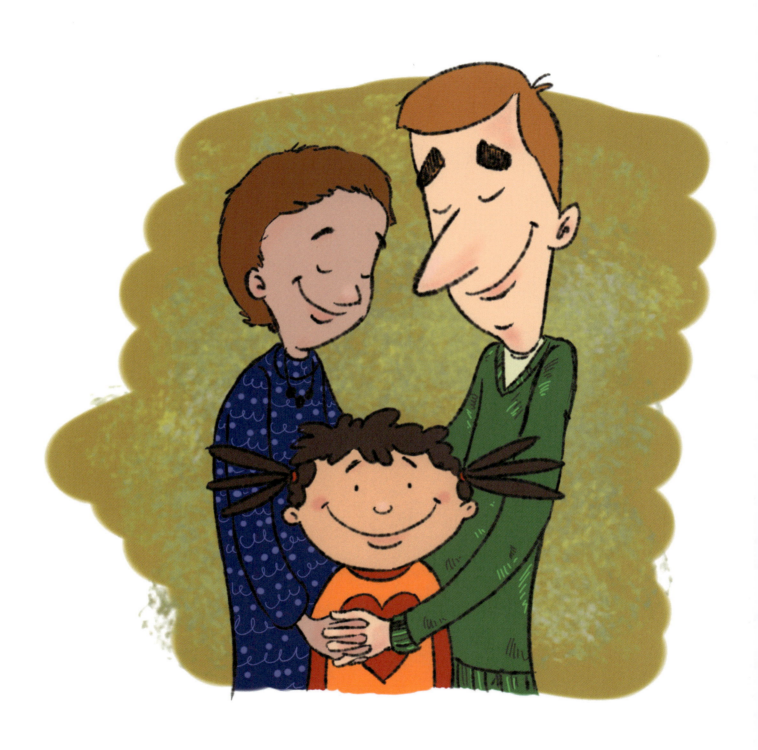

That would be amazing.

GLOSSARY

Here are kid-friendly explanations for terms used in this book, as well as for other words related to breast cancer. Remember, it's okay to say, "I don't know, but I'll find out."

Anaesthetic: Medicine that makes you fall asleep during surgery so you don't feel anything

Breast Cancer: Cancer that starts in the breast

Cancer: Unhealthy cells that don't grow the right way and spread or make lumps in your body

Cells: The tiny building-block parts of your body that change and grow all the time. Our bodies are made up of millions of cells

Chemotherapy (Chemo): A way to destroy cancer cells with medicine

Drains: After a breast cancer operation, some women need drains or tubes to remove lymphatic fluid from their bodies

Intravenous (I.V.): A way to give medicine through a needle into a vein

Lumpectomy: Breast surgery where the lump is removed but the rest of the breast remains

Lymphatic Fluid: A watery-looking liquid that travels around the body to help fight germs and infections

Lymph Nodes: Small parts of the body that clean (or filter) lymphatic fluid as it moves around the body

Lymphatic System: Tiny tubes that carry lymphatic fluid all around the body

Mastectomy: Surgery to remove the entire breast

Medical Oncologist: A doctor who decides what kinds of chemo medicines to use for cancer patients

Oncologist: A doctor who works with patients who have cancer

Operation (or Surgery): When doctors open up the body to try to fix it on the inside

Port (or Port-a-Cath): A little object placed under the skin so nurses and doctors can take blood and give needles without having to poke the skin every time

Radiation: A way to destroy cancer cells using energy rays

Radiation Oncologist: A doctor who decides what radiation treatments to use

Radiation Specialist: A person who sets up the radiation machine the way the radiation oncologist directs

Scar: A mark on your skin left by a cut or surgery

Surgeon: A doctor who does surgeries, or operations

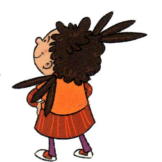

ACKNOWLEDGEMENTS

It took a community to get our family through my breast cancer treatments, and it took a community to create this book. Friends and family continually asked about the project, took care of my kids and offered contacts and information whenever possible. Every bit of support moved this book forward.

If breast cancer brought some darkness into my life, Rethink Breast Cancer showed me that light was still possible. Through their many programs for families and young women, I have found friendships, information and emotional support. I am so grateful to MJ DeCoteau, Farheen Beg and the Rethink team for having the vision of what this book could be and trusting me enough to try.

Many thanks to Morgan Livingstone, Child Life Specialist, who was a champion of the book from the moment it became an idea. Not only did Morgan help me explain the medical terms in words that kids would understand, but she made herself available to review the text, introduce me to contacts in the field as well as coming out on photo shoot days! Thank you to Jane Finlayson at Princess Margaret Hospital for welcoming us when we needed medical photographs. As well, the members of the #9 Writers Group always provided me with invaluable feedback and encouragement through the entire process. Thank you!

I was also fortunate enough to work with a few editors—all of whom came in to the project at the perfect moment. Shelley Hyndman got me on the right track from the beginning, Tanya Davies, Kim Thompson, and Erin O'Donovan all read and critiqued the various drafts I came up with, and Joan Hamilton graciously offered her expertise to make sure the content was relevant to women all across Canada. Finally, Katherine Dearlove worked through the final, careful edits before publishing. Thank you to all of you.

This book was created while three young children needed to go to school, hockey practices and music lessons. It would have been impossible without the help and support of many friends. In particular, I truly appreciate that Tania Richards cheerfully came every week to take care of our kids so I could lock myself away with my computer. Jim and Emily Stowe have also been tireless grandparents, constantly pitching in when we needed them.

And of course, my breast cancer peeps: Sarah, Heather, Jillian, Carol, Inez, Greer, Tasha, Kristina, Ingrid, Carmela, Maura, Kelly, Katherine, Victoria and Erin. These women never wanted to be in the position to review a book like this—but they did because they've been there. Thank you.

I met the illustrator, Jason Thompson, when our mutual friend Greer was diagnosed with breast cancer. I had dropped off my drafts for her to read, hoping it could be of help, but there were no pictures. At the same time, Jason had been working on illustrations for a similar book for Greer's daughters, but he didn't have any words. When Jason and I were later introduced by another mutual friend, we quickly realized we were both, quite literally, on the same page! I am humbled by Jason's commitment to bringing my words to life and also by his enthusiasm for the spirit of the project. He spent countless hours creating something far beyond what I could have envisioned or hoped for this book. When the photographer, Chris Gordaneer, joined the project and willingly devoted his time to produce the perfect shots, I was amazed at the professional calibre and goodwill that both Jason and Chris demonstrated. Thank you. Thank you. Thank you.

Finally, "thank you" does not seem enough for my husband, Erik. From the day I was diagnosed, he has held our family up beyond what I thought was possible. He continues to help me learn to embrace the life that I have, and to make it beautiful every day by filling it with friends and family. **-KS**

Thank you Karyn, for sharing your story and trusting me enough to help you tell it. Thank you to Willem Hart, for your sage counsel and thoughtful insights. Thanks, Leslie, for always being there. **-JT**

DRAW A PICTURE OF YOU AND YOUR MOM

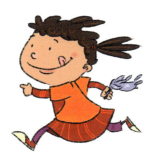

www.thekidsguidetocancer.com

CPSIA information can be obtained at www.ICGtesting.com
Printed in the USA
LVIW01n2216050516
486941LV00005B/19